EVERYONE wants a "miracle potion" that will melt fat away without exercise and without dieting. Most people are lazy and refuse to exercise. Some don't have the time and others can't exercise because of some debilitating illness.

And we all know that diets don't work, and we all agree that the only sure way to lose weight is to exercise and change our eating habits. But again, it's no fun to try to eat "right" all the time, to count calories, to read labels on everything we buy and to pass up the foods we truly enjoy. So, what is the answer?

CONGRATULATIONS! You have just found it! You have made one of the wisest choices in your life by buying this book because it has the answer to help you live healthier and happier in a more FAT FREE world.

Would You Like To . . .

LOSE
FAT
WHILE
YOU
SLEEP

No Dieting . . . No Drugs . . . No Exercise!

by

Pete Billac

Swan Publishing
Texas ❖ California ❖ New York

Author: Pete Billac
Editors: Cliff Evans, Dr. Chuck Galvin, Stuart Purcell
Cover Design: Sharon Davis

Other recent books by the author:
How Not To Be Lonely (for women)
How Not To Be Lonely . . . TONIGHT (for men)
New Father's Baby Guide
All About Cruises
Willie The Wisp
The Millionaires Are Coming

1st printing March 1998 -10,000
2nd printing April 1998 - 25,000
3rd printing May 1998 - 25,000
4th printing June 1998 - 15,000
5th printing July 1998 - 15,000
6th printing August 1998 - 25,000
7th printing (REVISED) September 1998 - 15,000
8th printing October 1998 - 15,000
9th printing December 1998 - 15,000
10th printing January 1999 - 50,000
11th printing May 1999 300,000

ALSO IN SPANISH

Copyright @ February 1998
Swan Publishing
Library of Congress Catalog Card #98-84047
ISBN# 0-943629-33-0

LOSE FAT WHILE YOU SLEEP, is available in quantity discounts through SWAN Publishing, 126 Live Oak, Alvin, TX 77511. Call at: (281) 388-2547, Fax (281) 585-3738 or e-mail: swanbooks@ghg.net
Printed in the United States of America

INTRODUCTION

I am an author and publisher. I also edit and ghost write. Counting everything, I have written, edited, ghost written and/or published somewhere between 400-500 books in my life. This book is probably *the* most important one I have ever written. Let me tell you why.

First, every book that I write or publish, my main goal is to help and/or entertain—preferably both. Being an altruist by nature, I want to help others. If, in my research, I find something that I determine is of great benefit to a vast majority, I rush to tell them about it. This is such a case.

Even as I write these words, my excitement is building; I truly can't wait to finish this book and get it to the world. I think I've uncovered a true **miracle solution** to making people live a healthier, therefore happier life.

Second, the manner in which this can be done is so simple, so easy, so logical that it benefits just about everyone. It is the absolute **easiest** as well as **effortless** way to rid your body of excess fat and lose inches. Getting rid of this excess fat helps the body to heal itself.

We'll only *touch* on diets; we all know by now that DIETS DON'T WORK! This is not a diet. This is a sensible, brilliant plan that allows you to do most of what you've been doing while you feel and look better and allow your body to help in the way nature intended.

DEDICATION

This book is dedicated to the memory of one of the nicest, sweetest, most brilliant, amazing, down-to-earth men I have ever met, **Dr. John H. Norris**.

John, in the short time we spent together, I learned to love you; all those who knew you did. I wish our book together would have become reality. Your untimely death has not completely soaked in yet. I still feel, that when the telephone rings at strange hours of the night, I'll hear your voice.

Now, you're in the house of the Lord. I know that He is happy with you. You sincerely and profoundly touched the lives of everyone who knew you. We all loved you and you will be greatly missed.

TABLE OF CONTENTS

What you are about to read in this book, in my opinion, is THE most amazing fat loss plan and product in the history of mankind. I have researched hundreds of claims on diet and weight loss plans, neither of which this is. We don't want to lose weight, we want to lose excess body FAT, therefore inches, resulting in a higher energy level and therefore becoming healthier. The body does wondrous repair on its own once we get this excess body fat out of its way.

Chapter 1

THE SECRET TO LOSING FAT

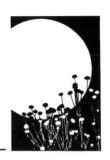

A close friend of mine, Dr. Robert M. Schwartz, wrote a book about 12 years ago titled, DIETS DON'T WORK. He followed that up about five years later with a book titled DIETS STILL DON'T WORK. Both became bestsellers. And why not? EVERYBODY wants to know how to lose weight and keep it off, but diets aren't the answer, are they?

In 1992 I received a manuscript from another friend, Lee Leva, who had been in the health club business most of his life. Lee came out with a product called FIT & SLENDER, a powdered drink, chocolate or vanilla flavor, which is superb. I still take it three of four times a week as a breakfast substitute. In it are a variety of vitamins and minerals. I mix it with water, diet cola, a little ice, vanilla yogurt and a banana. It's delicious.

For the fat burning ingredients in this drink to be the most effective, it is necessary to *exercise*. What's new, huh? We all know that exercise is essential to either become or remain strong and to tone our muscles. But what if we can't exercise? How about my friend who was stricken with polio in 1954? How can she exercise? What can she do about *burning off* fat?

And I have a host of lazy friends, don't you? Ones who just *don't believe* in exercise, or those too busy to take the time to exercise, and those who absolutely hate it. What is the answer for those who refuse to count calories and exercise? Do they just blow up bigger and bigger by the hour? Their blood pressure is soaring, as is their cholesterol, but they won't exercise or modify their eating habits until a doctor warns them that they'll die if they continue doing nothing.

About three years ago two medical doctors sent me a manuscript that I never published because it was written *by* doctors and *for* doctors, replete with medical terminology most people wouldn't understand. But, it caught my attention, and I read it carefully struggling through the "doctor" words. The words I did understand were *Behavior Modification*.

They advocated eating the *right* foods most of the time in order to lose weight and keep it off. No diet, you understand, and not doing without food, just eating in smaller portions and training yourself to be aware of and to avoid the foods with high sugar or oil content. And, of course, exercise.

They said to stay away from fried or greasy food, candy, ice cream and to count the grams of fat and count the calories in everything you eat. Who does that, huh?

It's just like using a juicer. You start with all the best intentions in the world but soon tire of a liquid diet. It's not fun feeding that noisy machine fruits and vegetables and especially cleaning it afterwards. And, you *might* be able to cultivate a taste for spinach, carrot and celery juice to where you don't gag as you drink it.

Sitting at a table for dinner with a large glass of green and yellow "stuff" is unappealing to every-one and the topic of conversation is usually cen-tered around the juice sipper who is not invited out to eat very often.

Dining out is fun. On most first dates, the agenda is dinner and a movie, right? I cannot recall ever reading a single line in a book or watch-ing a movie that said, "Let's diet and go to a movie." Meals are *social gatherings* of friends or family, where you eat and visit.

So, what do we have up to this point? Fit people who work out several hours a day at least three days a week who eat (or drink) foods that are no fun. We also have those who are depressed and eat and eat and eat and soon look as if they were blown up with Bavarian cream from their local donut shop. And don't forget those who have ever-expanding waistlines, hips, and thighs, that *no amount* of exercise will erase unless they adopt a regimen of eating the right foods and exercise for the rest of their lives.

Then, of course, there are those enviable ones who eat all they want and *never* gain weight. We never *really* get to like them, do we? They can just pig out at every meal and break all the culinary rules and keep their trim waistlines and enviable physique.

So, what *is* the answer? What can be done about high blood pressure, rising cholesterol level, always feeling tired, and our ever-increasing fat content? You might even *weigh* the same as you did in college, or when you were discharged from the armed services, or a year or so after you gave birth to that first or second child but that same weight has you wearing clothes that are larger than back then.

Let's face it! We are a lazy lot and why not? We are constantly enticed by televison with deli-cious food commercials that are downright sinful. Our highways are dotted by large signs sticking high into the sky that signal us to slow down and look at the absolutely beautiful color pictures of foods that are too appealing to pass up—and we can get this food quickly and eat it while we're driving.

STATISTICS and BODY FAT

Statistics say that we are losing the battle in the weight loss department because over ⅓ of all North Americans are overweight; 37.4 million of us are 35% or more overweight. We are, on the average, eight pounds heavier than we were 15 years ago!

It's been over 20 years since the fitness revolution began. We go to gyms, eat right, take supplements and spend over 40 billion dollars a year on weight loss and fitness, all to look and feel good. But, it isn't working. We still have a world mostly comprised of overweight people who could be healthier if they were able to get rid of that excess body fat.

Yes, look around at the people who are more than sightly to grossly overweight and if you ask, they will have a list of ailments to tell you about. Why? Because fat is unhealthy! Severely over-weight people run twice the risk of getting cancer, three times the risk of getting heart disease and up to forty times the risk of developing diabetes. And in some wild, crazy way we are losing not only our physical health but our emotional well-being. We carry around the burden of 10 or 15 extra pounds and pay the price with each bite of food. Why is this happening?

Well, it isn't entirely our fault. The *world* has changed and *we* must adapt. Our bodies were made to expend more calories throughout the day. Modern technology and our new more sedentary lifestyles have created this dilemma. We drive everywhere and rarely walk. It's gotten to the point where even walking holds many dangers.

If we want to walk around in the neighborhood, forget about a dog attacking; that's a past fear and now one of the least of our worries. We worry about getting hit by a stray bullet or some crazy person abducting us. Yes, the world has changed and we must learn to survive in it and EXCESS BODY FAT is a silent yet ever-present danger.

Because of this excess body fat we feel sluggish, we develop rheumatism-like symptoms, our cholesterol level rises, our blood pressure goes up, and our body doesn't have a chance to repair itself. So what do most of us do? We diet. Let's talk about diets for a moment.

DIETS

I am not going to attempt to "beat up" on all the diets, diet books, diet tapes, diet videos or diet doctors. I'm just going to appeal to your experience and logic.

With most diets, you are losing weight either by starvation or deprivation. Starvation means just eating less calories. Deprivation means choosing only specific food groups and eliminating others to change the way your body assimilates fat. In theory it works, but in the final outcome, the body gets its revenge.

Unless you adopt this diet forever, it just doesn't do you any good. Your body has become *accustomed* to what you have been eating for years and if you change it, the body balks. *Losing* weight is hardly the problem; *keeping it off IS!*

LOW CALORIE DIET

Just for the fun of it, let's explore a low-calorie diet. This is a diet specifically of starvation. Since you are changing the amount of available energy in terms of the intake of calories, your body immediately begins to look for other energy sources and since none are available, the body begins to convert the available carbohydrates that you have into energy instead of making protein like it's supposed to.

Having used up a lot of the body's carbohydrates, your body now begins to reduce the protein *synthesis* (the process of making a compound by joining together elements, simpler compounds or radicals) in order to conserve energy. The result is a LOSS OF BODY MASS! You are tickled pink. Who said a low-calorie diet doesn't work? But, this loss of weight is the loss of muscle, tendon and ligament as well as fat.

Next, your body begins to send you danger signals like fatigue, irritability, and loss of concentration. And then your friends (the ones who will tell you the truth) will say, "Gosh! You've lost weight—but you *look* terrible!" You know they are correct because you also *feel* terrible!

The next thing you do is abandon this low-calorie diet just to feel better. That's when your body shouts to you again. "It's about time," it says. "You lost 30% of our muscle mass and 50% of our reserves of energy."

So you eat more calories to rebuild what you lost but the *body automatically adds* a few extra pounds of reserve energy to prepare for another of your unwise decisions to diet.

LOW FAT DIET

You now want to try a diet that is low in fat. A sudden loss of fat means your dependency on carbohydrates and protein has to go up! You see, fat, carbohydrates and protein are staples of our existence, therefore a low-fat diet is one of deprivation!

Usable calories for energy comes from sugars that are stored in fat, so if fat is taken away, the body turns to the carbohydrates for its energy. Here is where you lose again. Let me explain.

When you restrict fat, your body begins to consume carbohydrates. By decreasing the carbohydrates, the body is forced to create more fat, which causes the body to increase fat accumulations. So in essence, a low-fat diet *makes* you fat!

LOW CARBOHYDRATE DIET

A low carbohydrate diet forces the body, in most cases, to conserve the fat energy it already has. Otherwise, it would have to begin using protein to make energy which is very inefficient for the body. Once the carbohydrates are at minimal levels, the body starts using the fat. Then, eventu-

turns to protein to retain the proper energy forces it needs, and you actually begin to **lose weight!** Good news, huh? Not quite.

Because, the loss of protein also **reduces the muscle mass** and the ability to rebuild and repair itself. So, what you're losing is muscle as well as fat and that is *not* a good idea. Let's try something else.

HIGH PROTEIN DIET

This is the **LEAST DESIRABLE** diet you can possibly go on! The theory is that it takes more caloric energy to digest protein than it takes to digest fat or carbohydrates. Therefore, you lose weight by burning more calories in the process of protein synthesis.

But, unless you have a rare body type that can deal with this extra protein metabolism, by increasing protein synthesis you produce an excess of *toxins* which can't get from the kidneys fast enough, and the result could be kidney stones, bad breath or *toxemia.* (Toxemia is a condition of blood poisoning, especially poisoning caused by bacteria transported through the bloodstream from a focus of infection.)

In plain words, ALL DIETS ARE HARMFUL

TO THE AVERAGE BODY if they starve or deprive the body of what's natural to it. In the last few decades, all sorts of diets have come on the market and they all claim to be "the" answer. If so, where are they now and why are we always trying new ones?

However, modern technology, along with Mother Nature, has given us the **solution** we have all been awaiting. It is a breakthrough in the weight/fat loss field. Let's talk about it because it might just change (or save) your life!

★★★★★★★★★★★★

On the following page is a *before and after* photo of Dr. Mark Evans. His testimonial is not as profound as thousands of others I have in my files, but I feel most can identify with Dr. Evans, those who need to lose just "some" weight.

"In 12 weeks I lost only 14 pounds, but **24 inches** overall; four from my waist alone. I tried various other weight-loss products and plans and NONE worked! I always gained the weight back.

"As a psychologist I've dealt with patients with weight challenges for years. This system has proven to be *the most* effective tool to provide physical/mental health intervention. It works on nearly everyone when it is followed correctly."

I questioned Mark on his photos. "Only 14 pounds Mark? It looks like about 40 pounds."

This is a perfect example where lean muscle replaced FAT. Look at the SIZE difference in his chest and stomach.

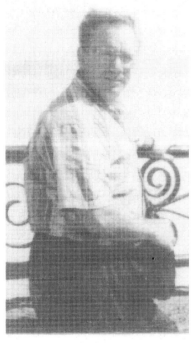 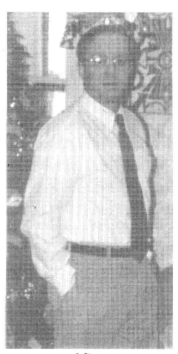

Before   *After*

Chapter 2

MIRACLE SOLUTION

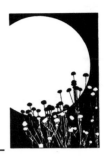

It was in the early 1980's, that Michel Grisé, a brilliant Canadian formulator, worked in the Veterinary Department of ABBOTT Laboratories in Montreal, Quebec, Canada. A veterinarian friend of his who worked for the Department of Agriculture of Canada asked him to formulate a food supplement to help reduce body fat in chickens!

Perhaps you've seen these egg-laying factories where hens are squeezed tightly in cages where they are fed and watered and remain in confinement until they can no longer produce eggs. These chickens couldn't exercise and they got fat and developed what is called *Fatty Liver Syndrome.* Their egg production lessened dramatically long before their egg-laying days were scheduled to be over.

It was impossible (certainly impractical) for these chickens to get exercise. There had to be a way to take the fat off so they would begin laying their normal supply of eggs without letting them out of these cages.

So they formulated a dry solution of additives and mixed them in with the chicken feed. Within five days, the body fat of the chickens was *reduced* and egg production went up! The Canadian beef, poultry, and dairy industries also experienced the same results with this formula. That's where the really *great* news begins.

Michel discovered that he was 30 pounds overweight and went to his doctor who put him on a 1,200 calorie a day diet. It didn't work. "This, of course, was an impossible task," Michel smiled. "I was traveling at least three days a week and had to eat hotel food. How can you eat but 1,200 calories in any one day? I was losing nothing." The doctor then suggested an 800 calorie a day diet.

"I decided that, due to the dramatic success of the product I used on the poultry, I would modify the formula by converting it from a powder to a liquid and test it on myself.

"By simply taking a tablespoonful of this new solution with a glass of water on an empty stomach each night just prior to going to sleep, I lost fat, weight, and gained more muscle tone. I lost 20 pounds in five weeks and two inches disappeared from my waist. I gained two inches across my shoulders. I did not exercise nor did I modify my eating habits!"

Michel then decided to offer the product to others. The results were spectacular. "This began in 1983. In the few years that followed," Michel added, "thousands of people lost fat and inches while preserving and building lean muscle mass. And up to this time, *tens of thousands* have experienced the same results." He named his discovery CALORAD.

With the help of an obesity specialist in Montreal, the first *clinical study* was conducted that consisted of testing 354 patients for 90 days. Neither their diet nor exercise patterns were changed.

The success rate of FAT LOSS was an outstanding 86%

HERE ARE THE ACTUAL FINDINGS

152 of the 354 tested had results in 1-30 days. (42%)
76 of the 354 tested had results in 30-60 days. (21½%)
77 of the 354 tested had results in 60-90 days. (22½%)
49 had little or no visible fat loss. (14%)

(There were benefits **other** than fat loss from this test. The testimonials is Chapter 3 will list some of them.)

HERE ARE THE SIMPLE INSTRUCTIONS

✔Take one tablespoon of CALORAD with eight fluid ounces of water on an EMPTY stomach just prior to sleep.

✔Your LAST meal should be at least three hours before taking Calorad.

✔No snacks or drinks other than water during those three hours prior to closing your eyes and going to sleep, not watching TV or reading, etc.

Does this sound too difficult for you? Remember, **NO DIETING and NO EXERCISE**.

Rena Davis, renowned clinical nutritionist, who in 1984 monitored 300 patients (ages 17 to 77) were given Calorad in her St. Helens, Oregon Clinic for a period of one year. These were **her** findings:

▶ The AVERAGE weight loss for one year was **9 pounds of FAT** and **3.75 inch loss per month.**

▶ Patients were not placed on a calorie restrictive

diet. (In other words, they ate what they had been eating prior to the study.)

▶ HYDROSTATIC (water) weighing was used to determine BODY FAT loss and LEAN MUSCLE MASS development.

▶ Patients were NOT required to exercise.

▶ 36% of the group gained LEAN muscle mass.

▶ Calorad was proven to be reliable and safe.

▶ The only side effects were POSITIVE ones.

Rena Davis took Calorad herself after having a child and lost 38 pounds. She reports her findings:

"These results were established over *13 years ago!* Since then, tens of thousands of people have achieved dramatic fitness and wellness results by using Calorad. Does this sound too good to be true? That's what I said before I reviewed the information and received the results for myself! The results have been phenomenal! It's too good not to share with you!"

THE PLAN

Take a (measuring) tablespoon of Calorad as is prescribed, and live your normal life. **That's it!** Do you understand? **THAT IS IT!** Calorad works while you sleep. Calorad works with or without the human will! Could it be any simpler? When you lose fat, you look great, as well as having more energy and stamina.

And, since fat is 2½ times as bulky as lean muscle mass, you lose **INCHES!** I know, this is just too easy, isn't it? And it is! I didn't believe it when I was first introduced to it but—**IT WORKS!**

UNDERSTANDING CALORAD

Many people will try *anything* to lose weight. So why not TRY Calorad? Calorad is phenomenal and will bring a healthier life to just about everyone who takes it. But Calorad can't do it all alone. It is **not** a license to eat an entire cheese cake or to go to one of those *all-you-can-eat* places until you feel you've gotten your moneys worth. It is merely a *better way of metabolizing your fat* the way nature intended.

For example, as children we produce large amounts of growth hormone which causes the body to convert and metabolize stored energy and produce muscle, tendon, and ligaments for growth.

As adults, growth hormone production slows, leaving us the option of using collagen instead to complete the same task. And, not *all* collagen products do the same job as Calorad does! Calorad is a formula *with* collagen as a primary ingredient. Let's now understand more about . . .

COLLAGEN

Collagen comes from animal products, usually beef connective tissues. Collagen is essential in the formation of strong muscle, tendon, ligaments, skin, nails, and hair. The **lack of collagen** causes the skin to hang, wrinkles to form, nails to break. A general body weakness develops simply because the body can't repair itself properly.

So, collagen is used in the protein synthesis to combine with the energy source—fat—to produce the necessary proteins that the body needs to repair these muscles, ligaments, and tendon. Now that we have collagen, let's find out how the body does the work.

Almost all body repair takes place during the *Alpha* phase of the brain's sleep cycle—the first several hours of sleep. The process involves the body shifting gears from the awakened *Beta* cycle of brain behavior that takes place during the day to a restful, rebuilding, rejuvenation behavior during sleep.

During this period of sleep, the body uses the available collagen and other vital nutrients and coverts them into new body materials. This process takes an enormous amount of caloric energy to complete and that's why one may wake up a few pounds lighter. What happens is an individual will *burn off* some calories by metabolism to make new body repairs during sleep. Therefore if one is deficient in collagen, you can't burn off the fat or repair the body very effectively.

Now, as wondrous as Calorad is, it is not to be used as a meal replacement; you need to eat three regular meals per day with the normal intake of 2,000 to 2,500 calories.

If you already exercise, there is no need to increase your exercise program since you'll be burning more calories by metabolism. But if you begin to exercise, or increase your exercise, *of course* it will have a faster effect on your body as any food would.

To assist your body in the removal of toxins and to work more efficiently, you should drink 8 to

10 glasses of plain water per day. Actually, you should be drinking this much water anyway regardless of the program. Water is the universal cleanser.

About a dozen years ago, a friend discouraged me from drinking iced tea with my meals because of the tannic acid in it; that it might give me gall stones or kidney stones. I didn't know if it was right or wrong but I listened; it's cheaper anyway. I know for certain that it changes—maybe improves—the taste of water.

One ounce of lemon juice (about the contents of one medium-sized squeezed lemon) supplies the body with 13 milligrams of vitamin C, about 22% of the RDA for adults.

Lemon in water is healthy; lemon is a neutralizer. It's involved in the pH balance in your body. So, skip the iced tea, the coffee, the coke, and drink water with some lemon in it.

Just before falling asleep, mix a **measuring tablespoon** of Calorad in an 8 oz glass of water and drink it. Remember that you want to catch the **beginning** of the Alpha cycle of your sleep. There's no need to put additional Calorad in your water. One measuring tablespoon is sufficient.

And, have an *empty stomach*. **Stop** all eating and drinking (other than water) at least three hours

BEFORE you take your Calorad in that glass of water (four hours if your digestive process is slow), after a full meal. If you had a salad or a light snack—two hours.

Finally, the entire program is based on a **3-month** plan. Everyone is different and personal results will vary. Besides, nature works best over time. Since it took many of you years to gain this body fat, it's ludicrous to expect it to just vanish overnight. We can't rush Mother Nature.

Remember, you are helping what the body does **naturally**. You are changing *metabolic function*, not going on a diet. DIETS DON'T WORK!

WHAT IS CALORAD?

Calorad is a *food* which has 14 calories; four grams of protein, zero grams of fat, and one gram of carbohydrate per one tablespoon serving. The collagen in Calorad is extracted from certified healthy bovine collagen. Each batch of collagen is inspected for purity by the Canadian government and additionally by private laboratory analysis.

Unlike any other collagen product on the market today, Calorad is the result of a **very specific extraction process** by Michel Grisé, the Canadian who created Calorad. Michel discovered a specific amino acid combination which is the key to Calorad's high success rate. Calorad does, in fact, have a certain *magic* to its formulation that many health practitioners describe as, "The most amazing nutritional supplement they have ever come across."

Calorad is being used by many consumers as a weight or inch-loss product. For those who carry around excess fat, it supports the building of **lean muscle tissue** which assists the body in burning sugar and fats more efficiently. Calorad does not stimulate, starve, or *trick* the body into weight loss. It does not require calorie counting, restricted diet, or exercise. This breakthrough formula feeds the body with a collagen-protein supplement resulting in the body shedding excess fat and toxins—**naturally!** Calorad supports lean muscle mass and facilitates FAT loss, consequently causing people to lose inches! Most lose a pant or dress size before they shed a single pound. Some will lose both weight and inches the first week, whereas others not until the end of the third month—and for some never.

Calorad, as I have previously stated, has a proven success rate. The formulation is designed to provide a highly bio-available fuel that each body utilizes according to its individual needs.

That's why not **all** Calorad users will see immediate results. The body may be using the collagen-derived amino acid components of Calorad to repair connective tissue damage of collagen disorders rather than using the product to facilitate an increased metabolism of fat or increased muscle building.

However, Calorad has demonstrated to have produced beneficial results on just about eight out of 10 of those who use it for 90 days. Test it for a month if you choose, but **three months** is the true test.

For those of you who are underweight or in good physical condition, Calorad assists the body in toning and can be used for increasing your energy level and stamina. Body builders and athletes are getting great results using Calorad before workouts. Consumers with a wide spectrum of health challenges are finding that this wellness formula is feeding the body with the perfect food for their needs.

Because Calorad is safe and effective, and **does not** require dangerous caloric restrictions, many chiropractic, naturopathic, and medical doctors are utilizing Calorad personally and professionally as a part of their total health program.

SIDE EFFECTS OF **CALORAD**®

One of the amazing **side effects** we've found is *weight loss*. Calorad®'s primary effect is to stimulate the body to rebuild muscle, tendon, and ligaments. And since the process does not interfere with any other bodily function, it has no effect on medications.

As a precautionary measure, pregnant or lactating women should not take Calorad®. And, consult a health care professional about Calorad® prior to administering to prepubescent children.

When you first take Calorad®, you might experience a slight weight GAIN! Why? Because muscle weighs more than fat and the conversion of fat to lean muscle mass can result in a temporary weight gain. But don't worry, it quickly reverses and goes in the other direction.

If you don't lose weight after the first 30 days, remember, the object is to **convert** fat into lean muscle. Your body might choose to change its appearance first. That's why I recommend that you judge Calorad® with a **tape measure**—by the way your clothes are now fitting—not a scale. The weight that begins to drop off will when it's good and ready and not before.

It's really about INCH LOSS and FEELING

BETTER. That's why I recommend a full **3-month program**.

Weight loss can sometimes be very sudden and quite dramatic. Still, don't worry. Your body is doing what is perfectly natural for itself. Unlike crash diets, losing fat to metabolism simply *uses* the fat and doesn't hurt the body.

THOSE WHO CAN NEVER LOSE WEIGHT

There are people who, no matter what they do, will NEVER lose weight. The reasons are. . .

✔You may have a malfunctioning thyroid gland. The thyroid gland controls ALL BODY METABOLISM. For those who suspect a thyroid problem, it's wise to have it checked and corrected by a physician *before* you begin any type of weight management program. When thyroid medication gets you under control, *then* resume Calorad®.

✔Due to the extensive use of antibiotics and drugs in this country, we have changed the natural body chemistry and flora of our intestinal tract. Therefore, all the **good and necessary** bacteria and microbes have been reduced, in some cases, destroyed all together. This has led to a silent infestation of YEAST, better known as *Candida Albicans*.

Candida is totally devastating to the body and only occurs when the body's good bacteria is no longer present to keep the yeast in check. Candida is commonly the cause of *vaginal yeast infections* or skin rashes, but the hidden effects are far more devastating.

Yeast coats the stomach, the intestine and other organs with a thick layer of mucus. This mucus coats the outer linings of the organs, and effectively stops the transfer of nutrients into and out of the body. Therefore, you take *in* food but *absorb* very little of it. The result is, you always *feel* hungry and, eventually, overeat causing further accumulations of excess fat.

Candida is a nightmare to get rid of. There is no medication that effectively eradicates Candida; it only controls it. If you have yeast in your system, it becomes very difficult to achieve good weight management. This means you'll not only never lose weight, but probably gain a few pounds per year no matter what you do.

But, there is an answer to **that** problem also. It is called . . .

AGRISEPT-L

Along with Calorad, Michel Grisé went one step farther and formulated Agrisept-L, a synergistic blend of natural **anti-viral, anti-bacterial, and antifungal properties** found in citrus. This biological formula was developed from the seeds of grapefruit, lemons and tangerines and helps to eliminate all non-wanted bacteria and microbes in the body.

It is nontoxic and has demonstrated in live blood cell testing to be helpful against the Candida Albicans outgrowth as a preventive treatment that subdues the fungus and assists the body on a weight loss program.

Agrisept-L addresses the problem of **CANDIDA**, as well as other inhibitors to weight loss including **HERPES, INFLUENZA, STREPTOCOCCUS, FUNGUS, PARASITES, STAPHYLOCOCCUS, SALMONELLA, ECOLI**, and **TOURISTA!** This natural product has NO harmful effects.

In an interview with Monsieur Grisé, I recall him mentioning that in the experimental stages of Agrisept-L, he put three liters (less than one gallon) of Agrisept-L into a **MILLION** gallons of *heavily polluted* water. "Within five hours, you could drink the water," he smiled.

YEAST TEST

The *amount* of yeast you have in your system will determine how quickly it can be removed. A quick way to determine how much yeast you have is to conduct a simple test.

Yeast can be detected in saliva. Put a glass of water on your night stand before retiring. First thing in the morning immediately upon arising (even before clearing your throat or brushing your teeth) is to gather some saliva in your mouth and *spit* it into the glass. Within minutes, if there is any yeast in your system, the saliva will immediately clump together and begin to "leak" down into the glass of water in tentacle-like fashion. It resembles a jellyfish if you've seen them under water.

If the saliva sinks down to the bottom of the glass quickly, you should consult a Health Professional to begin a cleansing program.

To **correct** Candida you could try 5 to 10 drops of AGRISEPT-L in juice or water twice a day just before meals until all signs of yeast are gone. Agrisept-L is somewhat bitter but in orange juice or apple juice, it is almost tasteless. I say stir it as you drink because it tends to settle on the bottom and that taste IS not pleasant.

Because you have signs of a yeast problem,

you may still take Calorad®. It has been proven that you **can** take Agrisept-L® while you are taking Calorad®, but take the Agrisept-L® with meals and make certain of the three hours with an empty stomach before you take the Calorad®.

As a **preventive** measure, add a few drops of Agrisept-L® into the juice of your choice before at least just one meal daily. Agrisept-L® has been laboratory tested with astounding results.

If there is NO YEAST in your system, the saliva will simply disburse on the top and not sink. Then, your Calorad® plan will work better.

CALORAD® ALSO HELPS BUILD MUSCLE

Athletes who want to BUILD their bodies for strength without using steroids or other harmful dietary aids can do it with Calorad®. The only **change** you have to make in this program is to take your Calorad® IN THE MORNING, in addition to at night. Take it one-half-hour before **beginning** your workout.

This way, you will build lean muscle mass and still lose fat because you are also taking it in the evening. Even then, you'll still enhance the building of your muscles, tendons, and ligaments.

OTHER POSSIBLE EFFECTS

Again, there are at least **2 million** Calorad® users; perhaps as many as 3,000,000. The few problems I ran across with friends who first began taking Calorad® were simple ones.

A mother of 60 and her two sons, ages 38 and 42, complained that the first few nights on Calorad® they each experienced slight stomach cramps. It was recommended that they take **half** the amount (one-half tablespoonful) in their eight ounces of water until the slight discomfort ceased.

It was explained to me by a physician that some people have this temporary discomfort because the body is flushing out toxins. The first night on a half dose, the discomfort ceased. By the sixth night they went back to taking the full table-spoonful of Calorad® without any problems. Soon, they lost inches and began to feel more strength and energy.

Another lady, in her early 60's, called about cramps in her lower abdomen the first two nights she was on Calorad®. Again, the half dosage was recommended. She still had slight cramps, but cut the dosage a bit more and in three days was back on the full program. I called her the following week and she feels an increase in energy and a lesser desire for food.

Several of my male friends, ages 35 to 55, reported an increase in urination during the first few nights of taking Calorad®. The same thing happened to me. Within a few days for all of us, this stopped and we all began sleeping more soundly. The reason for this was the sudden increase in protein into our bodies and we were (again) flushing out unwanted toxins.

Again, Calorad® is SAFE! Calorad® is an ALL NATURAL FOOD SUPPLEMENT that helps the body help itself!

*In this next segment are testimonials of those who used **Calorad®** from one to three months and longer. Their reports were edited only slightly to avoid duplication. If you read through them, chances are you'll find one that interests you particularly.*

Chapter 3

LIVING PROOF

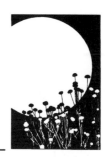

I know there are many questions you'd like to ask about Calorad that might pertain to your personal situation. These are in the chapter *following* this one. I wanted to put these testimonials here to really excite you.

As you know, I am not a medical doctor nor a nutritionist and, to be perfectly honest, I didn't believe it either. But it *sounded* so good, and it was too simple and too inexpensive **not** to try. Here is what happened to me and some friends of mine who began taking Calorad only six weeks ago.

My Experience:

For me, I slept soundly the first night I took Calorad for the first time in well over a year, and I continue to sleep soundly. I eat "right" most of the time, and *wrong* enough of the time to make eating fun. I take my breakfast malt three or four days a week and other mornings I eat bacon, eggs, buttered toast and I drink coffee with milk and two Sweet 'n Low packets; maybe two cups of coffee.

Sometimes I drink milk or orange juice instead.

I exercise a total of maybe 20 minutes every other day and I play golf three or four times a week—riding in a cart—and I drive as close as I am allowed to the ball to keep my golf etiquette intact. I am 5' 11¾" and weight about 183 pounds as a rule. When I started with Calorad I had "grown" to 191 pounds.

The second day on Calorad, I used a Body Fat Meter to measure my body fat. It showed 17.4% body fat. Within two weeks (still sleeping soundly each night and experiencing surprisingly other physical responses upon awakening that I can't specify), I lost 12 pounds in 14 days and my face became thinner and my stomach flatter. I lost an inch or two from my waist. I didn't measure prior to taking Calorad, I just *know* there's more room between my body and my pants at the waistline.

In the following two weeks I gained four pounds, but my appetite lessened; I now eat one full meal a day instead of two or three, and I'm never hungry. It's been three months now and the electronic Body Fat Meter showed 13% body fat! I'm told it isn't as accurate as the water weighing process. The fact is, I DON'T CARE! The same meter showed that my body fat went *down* more than 22% in 90 days. And, I **feel** terrific!

I had to travel for about ten days and didn't get a chance to exercise. When I went back to my exercise machine to do sit up presses, I glanced back at the weights thinking that my neighbor's teenage son had been using the machine and reduced the poundage. He hadn't! I added 20 pounds of weight and am now been doing three sets of 25 but with an increase of about 20% in strength. I can only attribute that strength gain to my taking Calorad® because the body DOES do miracles on its own when given a chance.

Your back just HAS to hurt less with less weight to carry around. I KNOW your ankles don't hurt as much with excess body fat gone—that's common sense, too. If you're carrying around a large stomach and thighs—say 20 or 30 pounds more than you need to, that's EXCESS baggage. That's like carrying around a packed suitcase all of the time. And what about your HEART when you carry around excess weight? It, too just has to work harder, now doesn't it? I don't claim that Calorad® REPAIRS your heart, just that the excess weight HAS to put a strain on it.

Calorad® is not a cure all—it builds LEAN muscle and lean muscle pushes away FAT. My analysis, only from a practical and not a medical standpoint, is that when the body GETS RID OF

EXCESS FAT it simply HAS to help us in a myriad of ways. That's common sense. You don't have to be a health practitioner or a genius to know that (as they say in Canada, ey?)

Without a doubt, the "good things" that have happened to me were after I began using Calorad®. I have more energy, my body weight has been right at 175 pounds and the sinus headaches I experienced often over the past 15 years have completely disappeared.

Perhaps it was just TIME for the headaches to be gone. And perhaps the "extra" strength I developed was just because it was TIME for me to get stronger. Or, maybe by ridding my body of excess body fat, these things happened. I don't mean to profess that Calorad® cures ANYTHING, but I feel it acts as a catalyst to help the body repair itself by getting rid of FAT!

After meeting with Michel Grisé at breakfast and having coffee with my meal, he asked that I use only *raw sugar:* "It assimilates better in the body and is much healthier for you." I also began drinking more water.

Another Couple:
My buddy, a 39-year-old golf pro, is about 40 pounds overweight. His name is Newton Pinkney

Hartline (we call him Pinkey) and he is the Director of Golf at Freeport Golf Club in Freeport, Texas.

The first night he took Calorad® and every night since, he slept soundly and felt rested in the morning. He lost 11 pounds in 14 days and inches from his blossoming waistline.

It's been three months now that he has been using Calorad®. He has lost a total of 26 pounds but he is eating *more!*

His wife, Carrie, is voluptuous (what you might call "stacked") and in the past 14 months since taking a job as a dental assistant, she gained 20 pounds. Within two weeks of being on Calorad®, she lost several inches from her **waist, hips** and **thighs** and REALLY looks great again. She says her sleep is much more restful and uninterrupted. She didn't weigh before she started and refuses to weigh now. She is happily losing inches.

It's now been three months on Calorad® for her, too. She went from a LARGE to a SMALL size in *Liz Claiborne* dresses and pant suits. Her only complaint is the cost of buying new (smaller) clothes and having to alter the ones she had been wearing. She is absolutely thrilled over this weight and inch loss and so is her husband, Pinkey.

Another friend:

Rudy Hebert is in his early fifties. About 30 years ago, Rudy was the 13th strongest man in the world in his weight class of 160 pounds. He now weighs about 200, and works out three days a week with weights but not on body building, just sessions to see how much he can still bench press, curl, jerk, etc. He was a total nonbelieiver.

"I'll try your *stuff* Pedro," (he told me after about three weeks of my badgering him) but you know I don't believe in it."

Within two weeks Rudy's bench press went up **25 pounds,** and he is thrilled. "My legs don't hurt any more and my torn shoulder feels better, I swear! I feel a lot better and I've lost a few inches from my waist."

This, I realize, is not something to make any of you run out and buy a bottle of Calorad®, but it really *is* something huge, if you knew Rudy. And 25 pounds when you are already bench pressing 300 is really awesome. When you press heavy weights, two or three pounds is a large increase. But to have 25 pounds all of a sudden "happen" is breathtaking to a lifter. He's had that increase in strength for about three weeks now.

The following are testimonials that I took from anywhere I could find them. I've met many of these people since, during my travels in promoting this book. Their lives have been changed because of Calorad® and so has mine.

Because of company policy and FDA rules they are not allowed to give specific testimonials on anyone but themselves, whereas I can. I do not work for the company or sell their products. I encourage everyone to use my book as a marketing tool because it is all TRUE and should I need to prove what I've written in a court of law, I'd welcome it (more publicity for the book).

Calorad® has proven to be a miracle for me, my family and many of my friends. I am devoting my life to bring this information to as much of the world as I am able. You see, Calorad® is not a drug, it is not a synthetic, it contains no stimulants; it is an ALL NATURAL food! It harms no one you can take it with any other vitamins or medication. It's a FOOD!

Before I had this book in print, I had given out Calorad® to over 90 people and received positive results on all but three individuals.

One used it for two weeks and quit. The other needs to lose 40 pounds, eats as if he's going to be electrocuted, and "manages" to devour a bowl of ice cream before bed. "Does this count as food?" he asks. Whew! No comment. The third one

is a golf buddy who (also) "took it once in a while."
What do they want, a **wish pill?**

TESTIMONIALS

☆ LOST WEIGHT
☆ LOST INCHES
☆ INCREASED ENERGY
☆ SLEPT SOUNDLY

ENTIRE FAMILY BENEFITS . . . .

"I hold a Doctorate in clinical nutrition,
specialize in preventive nutrition, and I'm involved
in Post Doctoral Research in nutrition at Ohio
State University. I fully researched Calorad®
through **Medline** and the **Internet** before I recommended it to friends and acquaintances.

"As a scientist and full time Cardiovascular
Research Consultant and Oncology Disease
Specialist working for a major pharmaceutical
company, I stay busy.

"I am an officer in the Marine Corps Reserve,
I serve as Executive Director to The Ohio Chapter
of the American College of Preventive Nutrition,

and am an active member of the Executive Board of Directors of the Franklin County Chapter of the American Heart Association (AHA), and volunteer for AHA committee.

"I personally have lost almost 12 pounds and over 2½ inches off my waist within my first four weeks on Calorad® and my wife Lynn lost three pounds and a total of five inches at the same time. I have increased energy and improved sleep.

"My wife previously suffered from frequent and rather severe bouts of insomnia, but now 'sleeps like a baby.' My teenage son and daughter also use the product and have seen weight loss and muscle toning as a result of their Calorad® use. My sister lost 10 pounds and two dress sizes in three weeks and loves the product."

Steven P. Petrosino, Ph.D., FACPN
Dublin, OH

PATIENTS LOST WEIGHT, INCREASED ENERGY . . .

"My Ph.D. is in clinical nutrition and I've been working in the nutritional field for 16 years. One of my principal focus areas is tracking people's health problems to their root as nutritional deficiencies.

From my broad experience researching health in relation to nutrition, I recognize Calorad® as a product that is positively needed by everyone, whether they have a weight problem or not.

"My experience with this product has been astounding. My patients, under less than ideal stress conditions, are losing weight and inches and gaining energy. Calorad® stimulates a source of natural energy in the body and those who are taking it are becoming self-evident testimonials to the power of this incredible wellness resource. There is no need to "try out" this product. It is an important source of nutrition for all bodies alike and it works. I would say it's the next universal juice drink."

Dr. Robert Fahey
Honolulu, HI

20 PATIENTS LOSE WEIGHT and INCHES . . . .

"I have been looking for a collagen-based product like Calorad® for over 20 years. I have repeatedly asked manufacturers to formulate a product like Calorad® to no avail. When I saw Calorad®'s ingredient set, I got in touch with a principal from the company. I checked the product out thoroughly and put 20 patients on the product. The success rate was incredible. I love Calorad® for a number of important reasons. "Firstly, this is a totally unique product. I know this because, besides my large professional practice, I have owned and operated four health food stores in the last 27 years. **There is nothing on the market like Calorad®**. I like the delivery system; it is simple and elegant. Without changing any major behaviors, my patients are losing weight and more importantly, inches.

"Beyond the weight management success, I believe that Calorad® supports people that are experiencing nutritional deficiencies. This is an important product for people who live in large cities and experience the toxicity endemic to urban populations.

"I have built a very large and extensive group of health practitioners and lay distributors. All this because I believe in the product and everyone sees the merit of the product almost immediately. My customers and my colleagues say 'yes' to Calorad®. I am pleased and amazed while doing well."

Dr. Ed Wagner, D.C.
Malibu, CA

LOST 14 POUNDS IN THREE WEEKS . . . .

"I work as a Registered Nurse and Hospital Administrator. My husband is a chiropractor. I started taking Calorad® on March 8, 1997. I was initially skeptical, but I've always said 'when they find something that will let me lose weight while I sleep that I would try it.' I did, and it worked. My husband is 6' 2" and went from 187 to 173 pounds in three weeks. I have lost eight pounds and 15 inches in four weeks and am still losing, but more slowly now. I am very happy we found Calorad®."

Kay White, MSN, RN
San Marcos, TX

CALORAD®'S POSTER GIRL OF NEW JERSEY. . . . .

"I had a weight problem but also a multitude of other ailments. I was catching cold after cold. Congestion made breathing difficult. I had allergy flare-ups, sinusitis, headaches, bloating, gas, heel spurs and weak nails. My triglycerides were up to 1,490 and cholesterol of 325. I had hot flashes, night sweats, and pre-menopausal problems. My bladder felt as if it wouldn't hold water anymore. At

53, I was a wreck! Janice Picking, my nutritionist, put me on Calorad® and Agrisept-L®.

"It's been a year now. I've dropped 40 pounds and numerous inches. My body looks as if has been re-sculpted. I have rid myself of all the conditions that were constantly aggravating me. My triglycerides are now 125 and my cholesterol dropped 100 points. I no longer need to take menopausal medication. I lost my double chin and the skin around my eyes has tightened. My upper arms have trimmed down and the cellulite behind my thighs is GONE! I sleep better and can handle stress. I have a brand new life!"

Evelyn Franks
Cape May, NJ

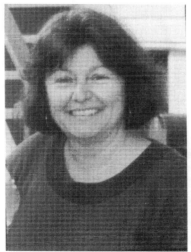
Before

I met Evelyn on a bus coming back from a convention in Orlando. She showed me her *before* and *after* photos which she proudly carries around, wouldn't you? Evelyn makes no medical claims about Calorad®, she just tells what happened to her once she started taking

Calorad® along with other changes she began to make such as *better eating habits* and wanting to become more active. I saw her again three months later and she still looks and says she feels TERRIFIC!

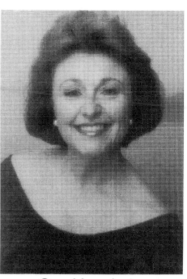

One Year Later

I talk to skeptics every day. One friend's wife said, "The **after** photo is a GLAMOUR shot!"

"Right," I agreed. "See if you can make that top photo look like the bottom with any camera in the world!" Gimmee a break!

SKEPTIC LOSES INCHES . . . .

My sister introduced me to this wonderful product after having me promise to take it for three months, reminding me that this extra weight did not just happen in a short time. Of course I was skeptical, but almost immediately I experienced an energy boost and deeper sleep but after one month there was no sign of weight or inch loss. By the end of my third month people began asking what I was doing because I lost 15 pounds and 15 inches.

Now, over a year has passed and I have lost a total of 35 pounds, 38 inches, my dress size shrunk from a 13/14 to a 7/8 and my waist from 36 inches to 24 inches. I did not have to change any of my eating habits or exercise and I feel terrific. My advice, don't be skeptical, it's easy to try and it works!

Carole Cadieux
Caledonia, Ontario

86% WHO TRY CALORAD® REPORT BENEFITS . . . . .

"As a licensed nutritionist and health food store owner with 30 years experience in the health and nutrition field, I feel confident that Calorad® is truly a unique and health-promoting product. Approximately 86% of our customers who try Calorad® are reporting benefits! I am also quite impressed with other nutritional support products in EYI's line and like the way they dovetail together in supporting the total health of the individual.

"My staff and I have shared Calorad® with others in the health care field and now have chiropractors, massage therapists, acupuncturists and others all distributing the product."

George Miller
Naples, FL

ENERGY, STAMINA & MUSCLE TONE FROM CALORAD®

"My results with Calorad® are phenomenal! Personally, I take it during the day for energy and stamina. I don't need to lose weight, but there's no denying the toning that's taking place in my body. My calves are harder and more defined, and my thighs are tighter. It's really quite remarkable.

"I've given Calorad® to many of my patients with tremendous success. One woman took off seven pounds in four days and is feeling noticeably more healthy and vibrant. A physician colleague of mine is seeing his abdomen muscles like never before and taking off pant sizes.

Dr. C. I. Middleton
Los Angeles, CA

SHANNON LOSES A COMPLETE PERSON . . . .

"In February of '97, I weighed 240 lbs. and was wearing a size 26 dress. I didn't believe in this *miracle potion* called Calorad® but I was more than desperate and I had to try it.

"In the first month, I lost only four pounds but I lost 10 dress sizes! After four months, I had lost

94 pounds and was wearing size 8 dresses!

"Now, I'm wearing a size four dress, looking and feeling great after losing 110 pounds and 22 dress sizes. Better yet, my skin doesn't sag after losing all that weight! Seeing is believing! Here's my before and after pictures."

Shannon Ellefson
Webb City, MO

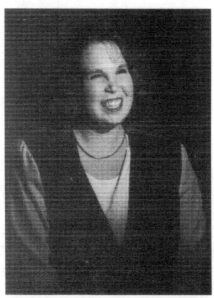

Before: 240 lbs. Size 26

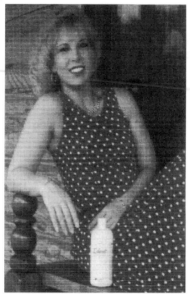

After: 130 lbs. Size 4

I had to ask her, "Are you sure you weigh 130? You look like you weigh much less." She quickly replied, "*Lean muscle mass weighs more! My dress size is four and I do weigh 130.*"

PERSONAL TRAINER TO WIN CHAMPIONSHIPS . . . . . .

A day in the life of Greg Sumner: Personal Trainer, Nutritional Consultant, National Power Lifting Champion with four world records, and the Silver Medal Champion in the Masters World

Championships. Here's the scoop on his first week of results with Calorad®:

". . . My first client of the day was Cheri Lerma who just won the State Power Lifting Championships, setting four state records. She seemed rather strong this particular morning. I passed it off figuring she might have had a few good meals and lots of rest. It was nothing compared to what my next client accomplished in her workout.

"We were doing a leg workout the previous week and it was a major ordeal to get the Power Lifting Belt to the first notch. I almost gave up but we finally combined our strength and did it.

"One week later she comes in weighing five pounds less and pulled the belt to the **second** notch all by herself and squatted 40 pounds more weight! I know she could have done more too! I was and am very impressed.

Greg Sumner
Seaside, OR

DRUG ADDICT GETS NEW LIFE . . . .

I was a drug addict since I was 11 years old. At he age of 31 a dramatic change occurred in my life but, unfortunately, a lot of damage had already been.

I was not able to eat much during the daytime and I had almost no energy. I drank a lot of coffee and at least a few liters of Coke every day.

After only two weeks on Calorad I cut back on my coffee about half and new energy had me finishing my chores earlier each day and I became more alert. I started craving fruits and vegetables and forgot about the Coke. People commented about my complexion clearing and the problems I had with pain from falling arches simply vanished. I also lost two pant sizes in less than a month. I praise God every day for the new life He has give me and thank Him for guiding me to Calorad.

Jackie Gervais
Carey, Manitoba

BODY BUILDER'S 3 P.M. ENERGY DIP GONE . . . .

"I am an avid body builder and have been paying attention to personal fitness as a passion for many years. I work out consistently, at least four times a week and am acutely aware of the way my body looks and feels. Since I've been taking Calorad®, I've noticed some tremendous changes in my physical well-being. For one, my energy level has evened out.

"My three o'clock dip has disappeared and I

feel consistently healthy and energized. As far as my external appearance goes, I'm seeing definition and toning that is new and extremely exciting for me. In the last few weeks I've been inundated with people from the gym and elsewhere asking me what I'm doing that's working so well! I'm very happy and more fit than ever. "

Bob Scullion
Los Angeles, CA

POLICE CAPTAIN LOSES 90 POUNDS . . . .

"I am a Captain in the CRIMINAL COURT DIVISION, responsible for the safety of 4,000 people each day. I am a 20-year veteran of the (New York Police) Force. I have personally lost 90 lbs. to date with the help of Calorad®. I take it twice a day, every day, and I am convinced Calorad® really works. I speak to anyone and everyone who will listen to me about the product."

Paul J. Christopher
Merrick, NY

LOST 22 POUNDS IN 11 WEEKS . . . .

"I've been a chiropractor for 20 years and have owned multiple chiropractic clinics. I was a pharmaceutical representative for over five years prior to becoming a chiropractor. I have not encountered a weight management product that comes even *close* to the effectiveness and wonderful results that are obtained with Calorad®. Personally, I lost 22 pounds in my first 11 weeks on Calorad®. I purposely ate all the foods I enjoyed and avoided exercise in order to prove the product. Boy, did it work!

"I lost four notches in my belt. My patients are getting very similar and wonderful results. I recommend every Chiropractor in the world to use Calorad® both professionally and personally."

Bill Uriarte, D.C.
Windsor, CA

AEROBICS INSTRUCTOR TRANSFORMS WITHOUT EXERCISE . . . .

"I am an aerobics instructor by trade. I didn't have any weight to lose by using Calorad® and was curious to see what this "muscle-builder" would do for my body. Well, in my second month of taking the product I'm noticing some incredible things. I do a lot of cardiovascular exercise but have not been lifting at all since I started Calorad®.

"Amazingly, my arms are now more defined than they were when I was lifting weights. I'm starting to see cuts in my leg muscles that have never come to the surface before. Just the other day, I visited my massage therapist who has supported me as an athlete for ten years. He could not believe the enormous change in my body's muscle composition.

"He was blown away that the body he had been working on for 10 years had changed so magnificently in just over a month. He wanted to know what I was doing and bought two bottles of Calorad® immediately. I didn't know that I could feel better and stronger, but Calorad® has changed my life in some pretty significant ways."

Karla Yates
San Fernando, CA

FITNESS TRAINER LOSES INCHES FROM WAIST . . . .

"I am the owner and operator of *Executive Mobile Fitness.* My gift in life has been to train personally and to educate properly in all facets of exercise, personalized fitness training programs, and health & wellness. I've been taking Calorad® for four months and am experiencing increased cardiovascular fitness and substantial increases in the weight I lift. I have lost **nine pounds** of **body fat,** gained nine pounds of muscle back (per my body composition machine) and lost three and one-half inches off my waist line.

"My most dramatic physical changes have been three inches of muscle growth on my chest and back. Calorad® is a tremendous product! I recommend it to my clients and everyone I meet!"

Michael Paul, N.A.S.M.C.P.T.
Lancaster, CA

DESIGNER GETS AMAZING RESULTS WITH CALORAD®

"I started taking Calorad® around the end of last September when a client of mine, Cheryl Ward, brought it to my attention. Immediately, people saw that I was losing weight. I didn't see it, but they did. Toward the end of my second bottle, I realized I was actually shrinking before my own eyes. By the end of the third bottle I had lost four inches off my waist, four inches off my hips. I was a totally transformed woman. I looked like a new person. I've been a designer for 20 years.

"My clients, who hadn't seen me in a while, started asking what was going on. In designing clothes for celebrities it was just a natural to help them find a way to look better in the clothes I designed for them. Before I looked up, to my surprise, I had sold 20 bottles. My husband, Jonathan, and I are building a terrific business with lots of wonderful friends. What a blessing this product is in our lives."

Angela Dean
Clothing Designer
Los Angeles, CA

WEIGHT + INCHES = BELIEF . . . .

There is a history of health problems in my family, all stemming from being overweight. In September 1998 I weighed 240 pounds with a 42" waist. After taking Calorad® for only 18 days I lost

20 pounds and my waist went to a 38. The next 57 days I dropped 35 **more** pounds and 2 more inches of my waist. My goal is to be 175 with a 32" waist. Many of my family members are now on the product and they have ALL experienced almost miracle results. Calorad® is bring a happier and healthier life to me and the ones I love. I'm so thrilled that I became involved in the business because I truly want to help others.

Tim Blacklock
Kingston, Ontario

LOST 10 POUNDS AND RAISED HER TUSH . . . .

"I planned to have to spend the rest of my life looking like a fat little Jewish grandmother. It's certainly not what I dreamed of for myself and the vision, quite frankly, made me very sad. Three weeks ago I started on Calorad®, pretty desperate for something to work out for me. Within a matter of three days I could feel a shift taking place. In three weeks I've taken off 10 pounds without changing a thing in my life. My legs don't rub together, my arms don't pudge out, my stomach has gone down two inches and my tush has raised up. I never thought this could happen to me. It is beyond a dream come true."

Ava Gudeman
Los Angeles, CA

SIZE TWENTY TO SIZE TEN . . . .

"I have had phenomenal results with the Calorad®. When I started taking it, I was wearing a size 20. While on my second bottle, I went to the store to buy a new pair of jeans and discovered I could fit into a size 16! I lost 50 pounds in my first four months and went from a size 20 to a size 12. The next four months I lost an additional 16 pounds and continued losing inches. Today, I have lost a total of 64 pounds and am sporting a size 10 wardrobe, looking and feeling fabulous!"

Linda Jones
Spokane, WA

EX-DIETER LOSES 40 INCHES IN FOUR WEEKS . . . .

"I've done every diet that comes along, rice diets, high protein diets, straight vegetable diets, you name it, I tried it. I started taking Calorad® and as of four weeks now, I have lost 15 lbs. and more than 40 inches all over my body, five inches in my abdomen, and five inches in my waist! I drink 80 ounces of water a day, approximately 2½ quarts, which I believe, along with the Calorad®, is the winning combination. I was going into X-large sizes. Now I can easily fit into size 14. I think Calorad® is the greatest thing going!"

Judy Andrejski
Bay City, MI

BUFFY'S WEARING A DRESS THAT HASN'T FIT IN TEN YEARS . . . .

"I have been battling fat all my life and losing the battle. On November 26, 1996, I first started on Calorad®. I traveled to Florida over Christmas and New Years and put it to the test. This was the first time in 17 years that I didn't gain weight during the winter months. Since starting Calorad® I have lost 24 lbs. and 20 inches. I started out in a size 20 and now I'm a size 16. I don't have to shop for clothes in the "plus size" stores anymore!

"I am the mother of four and I feel like I'm 20

years old again. I am still going strong at midnight. The *carpel tunnel syndrome* I've had for 15 years is gone. I sleep soundly and wake up refreshed. I wore a dress to church that I haven't been able to fit into for 10 years. I got so many compliments. It was a wonderful feeling! I feel like I have control over where I am going for the first time in my life!"

Buffy Kasinec
Elyria, OH

MARINE HAS BEST ABS EVER AFTER TWO WEEKS . . .

"I'm a massage therapist and a former Marine physical fitness instructor. I did sit-ups with 50 pounds behind my neck. You could kick me in the stomach and it wouldn't hurt me, but you couldn't see abs. After two weeks on Calorad®, my abs are cut better than they've been in my whole life! It's been 10 weeks now and I've gone from 173 to 160 on the scales and lost two inches in my waist. I'm training less, yet my leg muscles are more defined and I'm looking better than I have in a long time!"

Scott Stafford
Lewisberry, PA

FIGURE RESHAPED IN 30 DAYS . . . .

In June of 1996, I began taking Calorad® to lose five to ten pounds. I experienced a two to three pound weight loss in the first 30 days, and I noticed my skin starting to improve, and a general feeling of well-being.

In the following month, my clothes began getting looser in the waist, hips and thighs as I had lost about two and a half inches overall. My total weight loss is about seven pounds now and one size smaller in my clothes.

I'm thrilled with this and continue to see a muscle tightening and reshaping of my figure. I am now within my ideal weight range and will continue taking Calorad® for the rejuvenation I see and feel week by week.

Sabrina Dancy
Lake City, FL

LOST 15 POUNDS IN SIX TO SEVEN WEEKS . . . .

"I opened a retail store and have been operating it for four years now. I sell herbs, teas, vitamins, minerals, homeopathic products, books, and specialize in wellness and cleansing. Many people were coming in and asking, 'What do you have for weight loss?' So, I bought five bottles of Calorad®, used one on myself and lost 15 pounds in six weeks.

"When Calorad® began working for me, I decided to write an article for the Health and Fitness page of our local paper. People started calling the newspaper to find out about Calorad® because they didn't know how to reach me. I had to pick up 36 bottles, 18 of which went out of the store in one day and I had people on a waiting list. I then had to close the store and put up a sign, 'Sorry, had to go to Santa Monica to pick up Calorad®!'

"But that was only the beginning! The results have continued to fire up the demand. Today, I have a sign on the street outside my store that reads, *Lose Weight While You're Sleeping.* That draws people in and I give them a brochure and talk with them about Calorad®. I can never stock enough Calorad®."

Cathy Richer
Health Food Store Owner
Fallbrook, CA

HEALTH FOOD STORE MANAGER LOST 10 LBS. IN
THREE WEEKS . . . .

"I currently manage a health food store that began offering Calorad® to our retail customers three weeks ago. Already we have sold 140 bottles with over 25 people on a waiting list for the next shipment! I've been in the health field for 25 years and watched products come and go. I really like Calorad® because it contains no stimulants, no suppressants, has no side effects, and everybody can use it. In fact, I am impressed with the other products in the EYI line as well. Grapefruit Seed Extract has always worked well but it seems that the added citrus extracts in Agrisept-L® may make it an even better formula.

"I have personally been on the product for three weeks now and have lost 10 pounds and 1½ inches around my waist. I also lost my craving for sweets. I feel so good and have so much energy that I went out and joined a gym. I am very pleased with Calorad® to say the least!"

Jim Wilk
Health Food Store Manager
Lansdale, PA

✶✶✶✶✶✶✶✶✶✶✶✶

Has this been exciting? Even after reading all of this there are skeptics but please, maybe for the first time in your life, take a chance to lose fat, feel and look better and **actually *be* healthier.**

We didn't PAY these people to give their testimonials; they volunteered them. And Calorad® has been around a long time and is here to stay. It's worked wonders on so very many people and made their lives so very much better. Try it on yourself, please!

Also remember, LOSING FAT is a *side effect* from using Calorad®. My personal experience, and from interviewing hundreds who are taking the product, is your ENERGY LEVEL will increase almost instantly. From this, you automatically become more active and it *does* make you aware of eating more of the "right" foods, drinking more water, and staying away from the constant eating of "bad" foods, thus helping the entire plan work.

I still interview people who are on Calorad® and I am constantly amazed at their results. It makes my life more fulfilling because I am a part of letting others know about this wondrous miracle that takes away INCHES and FAT. And, when your body loses fat, it repairs many ills.

And ladies, woefully, it seems to work faster on men, but regardless of your gender, Calorad® will do wonders for the way you *feel*. If you are one of the overFAT, be patient. Remember, it took you years to get this way so give Calorad® time to work.

I must have a few THOUSAND testimonials that are sent to me and more often than not, when I hear the wonders it's performed on so many, tears of joy well in my eyes. I feel good about myself. Being involved with Calorad® has helped me physically, mentally, spiritually and if I sell as many books as I anticipate, financially as well.

Chapter 4

FREQUENTLY ASKED
QUESTIONS

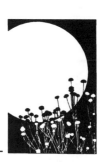

Q. What is Calorad®?

A. Calorad® is a food as well as a product for weight management. It's collagen formula supports the body in building lean muscle tissue. For those who carry around excess weight, the building of lean muscle tissue assists the body in utilizing sugars and fats more efficiently. For those who are trim and don't need to lose weight, Calorad® supports the body in building strength and vitality.

Q. Is Calorad® FDA approved?

A. There is no need. It is a food supplement. No synthetics, no chemicals, no drugs, no stimulants; only protein, which is a food.

Is it patented?

A. No! And that is a bright question. Michel Grisé neither needed nor wanted a patent. His formula is secret and others have tried to duplicate it but could not. Coca Cola isn't patented either.

Q. I'm about 20 pounds overweight but my sister is trim. Should I take Calorad® and forget about her?

A. Calorad® is good for **all** body types. It's a *food supplement*, specifically a *collagen* supplement, that enhances the body's natural mechanism of rejuvenation and repair. Everyone benefits from Calorad®.

 Why does Calorad® work?

A. These are medical facts: When we go to sleep at night, the first 45 to 90 minutes of sleep are a period of productivity in the body. Our minds go to rest, but our bodies go to work in a process of revitalization and repair. Calorad®, when taken on a stomach empty of food for at least three hours with a glass of water directly before sleep, fuels and feeds that process. Just like any protein that builds the body, Calorad® builds in a heightened way when taken in this manner.

Q. Will I have to diet and begin (or increase) my exercise schedule?

A. **No and No!** The beauty of the program is that it is so simple. The cessation of food intake **three hours prior to sleep**, if not being done already, is the only stipulation, which in and of itself is a very healthy behavioral shift.

And, there's no need to diet. In most diets, 30% of your muscle mass is sacrificed for weight loss. With Calorad®, the **building** of muscle is what causes the weight reduction, consequently, people lose inches as well as pounds. Remember, diet is *what* you eat, not *how much* you eat. So please eat healthy foods.

As far as exercise, do as little or as much as you were doing before you found Calorad®. My personal experience is that the increased energy from taking Calorad® should make you WANT to do more physical activities.

Q. How much weight will I lose?

A. That's hard to tell. Many people lose *inches* before they ever lose a pound, their clothes fit different or perhaps they drop a dress/pant size without noticing any changes on the scale. Then, there are those who initially **put on** weight, but **lose inches** because muscle weighs almost **twice** as much as fat.

Q. How can I be assured that it will work on me and I'll lose fat?

A. **You can't!** You can only give it a trial. However, it works in positive ways on just about everyone judging from the testimonials. The results show up differently in each subjective body. Some will experience noticeable results in the first week and some not until the third month. Some will lose steadily at a very slow rate (for instance one pound every two weeks) and some will plateau out for a while and for others, fat just seems to melt away. Remember, the **trial period** is 90 days! Trust me, it's worth the time.

| Q. | What else does Calorad® do? |

| A. | I can only tell you to go back through the many testimonials of what others claim |

happened to them once they began using Calorad®.

In my interview with Michel Grisé, he pointed out to me how your skin becomes more elastic once it's sagged from age or weight. I talked with others who claim their age spots disappeared, of wrinkles vanishing, and even those who believed their hair grew.

At a meeting, one lady said she feared she would be totally bald, because her hair was falling out in clumps. "Within six weeks after beginning to use Calorad®, it came back—but it was gray. I can dye it," she said. "I'm just so thrilled that its coming back regardless of the color."

I am not saying that Calorad® will **grow hair!** In consulting with physicians, their explanation was that the lady apparently had a medical problem that her body corrected once the excess body fat was gone.

Q. Suppose it doesn't work on me at all?

A. For those 14% who do not experience any weight or fat loss, this could be due to latent thyroid problems, mineral deficiency, colon health, or personal chemistry. See a health practitioner to get these problems resolved, and *then* give Calorad® a 90-day trial. It could change your life!

You will *still* benefit from the ingredients in Calorad® much in the same way you benefit from taking vitamin or mineral supplements. There is **no** *wrong* **experience** from the product. It is simply life supporting in various ways for different people.

Q. How do I take Calorad® for *optimum* weight management results?

A. As mentioned several times earlier in this book, one tablespoonful of Calorad® should be taken directly before sleep, at least three hours after your last meal, with a full, eight ounce glass of water. If you have a *heavy* meal (steak and potatoes) make if **4** hours, regular meal—3 hours, and a salad or snack, two hours. You can mix it with water or drink them separately.

Don't take vitamins, an antacid tablet, even

a PILL—NOTHING but water—three hours prior to taking Calorad .You see, if there IS acid in your stomach, it tends to absorb the Calorad® and renders the protein amino acids useless. DO IT CORRECTLY for the best results.

Do NOT put Calorad® in the refrigerator; it needs to be taken at room temperature otherwise the stomach has to warm it with acid that will lessen the effectiveness of Calorad®. Now, I put it in the fridge and it worked wonders on me. But experts tell me to keep it at room temperature.

It is also healthier to **drink eight to ten glasses of water each day** to help cleanse your system. Too, adopt smart eating habits, and avoid fat-causing foods as much as possible.

Remember, if you plan to read or watch television in bed, **wait** to take Calorad® until you **finish** those activities. Calorad® works best if the stomach is empty of food for at least three hours and you should take it just as your head hits the pillow.

Q. How do I take Calorad® for energy and stamina?

A. Calorad® works to sustain daytime energy levels when taken in the above "nighttime" manner. But, for endurance and stamina, Calorad® can also be taken during the day approximately **one half hour** before meals. Athletes can take Calorad® 30 to 45 minutes before working out to support endurance and strength.

One friend of mine, a power lifter named Rudy Hebert, whom I mentioned earlier (who had to be convinced to take Calorad®—no, I *badgered* him, remember, but only because I cared) is now shouting Calorad®'s praises all over Texas and Louisiana because he was bench pressing about 8% more after being on Calorad® only two weeks.

He said he had been stuck on a certain weight for over five years prior to this before taking Calorad and he became TWENTY FIVE POUNDS (8%) stronger. And, 8% is a *lot* when you get up into the hundreds of pounds.

Q. How should I take Calorad® if I don't want to take off weight?

A. Calorad® is a *nutritional supplement*. Those individuals who need to lose excess pounds and inches experience these results with Calorad® because it supports the body in building muscle mass and, consequently utilizes fats and sugars *more efficiently*. Calorad® is not exclusively for any one body type, however. It can be taken by **all** physical types alike as a strength optimizer and nutritional support product. For individuals taking Calorad® as a nutritional supplement, any of the above methods are appropriate for usage.

Q. Can I take Calorad® if I'm taking other vitamins and minerals? How about if I'm on medication?

A. **Yes and Yes!** Calorad® works with virtually *all* other nutritional supplements; that's the great part. However, it is suggested that if you take other nutritional supplements, take them with your **last meal** to maximize the efficacy of Calorad®. Calorad® works best when there is no other activity in the digestive system. Remember, drink water, water, water.

Similarly, if you have any questions about the compatibility of your medication with Calorad®, it is suggested you take a bottle of Calorad® with you to a health practitioner before proceeding.

Q. What if I don't lose any weight the first 30 days on Calorad®?

A. That happened with three of the people I sold a single bottle of Calorad® to. One friend at Hillcrest Golf Club, Joe DeJongh, took a bottle to lose weight. I had been using Calorad® for two weeks when I mentioned it to him. I had lost 12 pounds so I was a believer.

I called Joe about 25 days after he began taking Calorad® to find out what he had lost. "The price I paid for that stuff," Joe replied, laughing. "But I sleep better and I feel better." The **true test** is **90** days.

Q. NOW for the BIG QUESTIONS. WHERE do I get Calorad® and is it expensive?

A. Calorad® is not sold in ANY large retail stores; it is sold mostly through a network of over 325,000 independent distributors and small business owners. The chances are, it can be purchased in the very city or country in which you live. And, the price is less than a dinner for two at a nice restaurant. It varies between countries.

Where you can get it is easy. Hopefully, there will be sticker in the back of the book with the name and number of an independent distributor. If not, call the publishing company and, as a special service to those who sell and to those who want to take the product, we'll put you in touch with someone near you.

Q. For those that Calorad® does NOT work on, what is their option?

A. Excellent question. I've been traveling across the country and into Canada for about 10 months now and I DO, in fact, meet and hear of those that Calorad® has no VISIBLE effects on. Let me share this with you.

The major reason people see little effect with Calorad® is COMPLIANCE; they want to do it THEIR way. It doesn't work YOUR way, it works OUR WAY! You cannot take it with orange juice; take it with 7-8 ounces of WATER, preferably *distilled* water. You cannot get benefit from it if you snack on popcorn, take a Rolaids or vitamins or any other pill within THREE HOURS of taking Calorad® and going DIRECTLY to bed.

The #2 reason it might not be causing you to lose fat if that you have a YEAST problem. Rid yourself of yeast (candida albicans) with Agrisept.

The #3 reason is THYROID problems; have your doctor arrest your thyroid condition BEFORE taking Calorad®.

The #4 is that you have PARASITES. Don't

panic! EVERYONE has parasites and you get rid of them today and you'll get more tomorrow.

Again, I'm not a medical person nor a health practitioner, just a writer who investigated a phenomenal product and plan to spend most of the rest of my life telling others about it—because I care and I CAN make a difference.

To go into parasites would be cheating you; all I know is that there are parasites and there are BAD parasites. You, on your own, find out about parasites from any health practitioner. If you CARE about your body, about losing FAT, about feeling healthier, DO THE RESEARCH.

The last reason (I'm told) is that if a woman has recently given birth to a child, she might be suffering from a CALCIUM deficiency so fortify yourself with calcium. Again, ask a health practitioner about it. If you bought this book through an independent distributor of EYI, ask THEM and have THEM find out for you. They'll be pleased that you asked.

But, GOOD NEWS! EYI has now come on the market with Calorad®AM which was formulated to work better on those with a LOT of weight to lose as well as those who have not experienced sufficient fat and inch loss they expected from Calorad®.

What I'd like you to be acutely aware of, is that you might not be able to **read** any weight loss on your scale, but look for the INCH loss and how you FEEL. As I candidly describe in many interviews when telling about Calorad®, it tends to GREASE RUSTED SPRINGS. When people out of shape and/or over 50 first get up in the morning, they might hear a *snap, crackle* and *pop* when they take a few steps. It's the lack of collagen that has leaked from their body over the years which Calorad® replaces.

It's the added **energy** you get from Calorad® too, as well as the fact that it IS forcing fat from your body by building lean muscle mass. Those who know what they're talking about tell me that when you rid the body of excess FAT, it does miracles on its on.

I don't feel that Calorad® is a miracle CURE for anything, other than supplying your body with collagen and building lean muscle. I think it's your BODY that does the curing. Calorad® just acts as a sort of *buddy* who pushes you out the door on your first parachute jump so you won't wimp out at the last minute. I feel it's the catalyst that gets all this "stuff" in motion.

Something else: Different people and companies are advertising a product "like" Calorad®

that costs less. They say that they can sell you a collagen based product for less money and that their formula is the SAME as the label on Calorad®.

,   May be. The problem I have with that is that they aren't AWARE of the FORMULATION of Calorad®. The formulator, Michele Grise doesn't LIST the amounts or the formulation of the fat-burning amino acids in Calorad®. So, NOBODY knows and NOBODY has been able to copy the formula. Calorad® is UNIQUE and Calorad® WORKS!

I've been sent and bought some of the products "out there" and it has NOT worked on me and several of my "test cases". The truth is, I WANTED it to work because my *mission* it to help people. And, if I can help them CHEAPER, I'd do it because then I could help more.

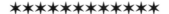

Chapter 5

CALORAD® FOR PETS

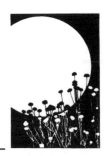

"Products that sound too good to be true usually are. Calorad® is an exception. It is the only product I have actively endorsed during my 28 years as a veterinarian. I have seen with my own eyes what this amazing nutrient can do. It is, without question, much more than a safe and effective weight loss product—it is a total body wellness supplement!

"I now have approximately 500 dogs, cats, and birds as well as over 500 pet owners and their friends on Calorad®. It is a great source of satisfaction for me to hear from people every single day that they are benefitting from the product or that their pets are. Animals become rejuvenated; i.e. dogs start acting like puppies after being on Calorad® from one day to three weeks.

"I have found the Calorad® supplement to be very useful in treating the older pet who is slowing down, sleeping a lot, and doesn't have as much enthusiasm. I also recommend Calorad® for the middle aged, active pets to maintain their health, staying playful, active and out of pain.

"Pets have a shorter life span than humans

and I believe Calorad® can help postpone the inevitable deterioration of these pets as long as possible.

"A Golden Treat® supplement (with Calorad® in it) can improve many health situations including:

✔ counteracting the signs of aging
✔ increasing coat luster
✔ aiding in weight reduction
✔ pets with slipped disks
✔ improving energy levels
✔ any pet exhibiting slow healing
✔ recovering from serious injury
✔ recovering from surgery or illnesses
✔ maintaining youthful qualities such as playfulness
✔ improving mobility
✔ slowing down joint degeneration in arthritic pets
✔ slowing down or reversing muscle atrophy and weakness
✔ helping pets with fatty livers or elevated blood fat levels
✔ lowering blood sugars in diabetic pets
✔ helping pets along with thyroid problems
✔ reducing fatty tumors in pets
✔ minimizing the side effects cortisone therapy
✔ improving weak muscles and thin skin
✔ helping the normal healthy pet maintain overall wellness

Prevention is better than cure!

Chuck Galvin, D.V.M.
Novato, CA

DISCLAIMER

As the author, I mention several times in this book that I am neither a physician nor a health professional of any kind; I am simply a writer who came across an amazing product that I want to share with mankind.

This book is in its 10th printing in nine months. In traveling the US and Canada promoting the book, I have thousands of testimonials from those whose lives have changed for the better because of Calorad® and the many other amazing products from Essentially Yours Industries.

Much of the information in this text is from my active and extensive research. I solicited the aid of health practitioners, physicians, nutritionists, chiropractors, pharmacists and from interviews with the brilliant man who formulated Calorad® as well as from testing on myself—personally, my relatives and friends. The results are phenomenal!

I work closely with most of the field leaders. I believe so fervently in their conviction to help others that I plan to devote years of my life telling about Calorad® to anyone who will listen. You see, I've witnessed the miracles Calorad® has performed. Look at page 20 (Dr. Mark Evans), page 53-54 (Evelyn Franks), and page 57-58 (Shannon Ellefson) and see for yourself!

No one in Essentially Yours Industries, in any form or fashion, are to be held responsible for whatever I've written in this book but without their assistance I would have had little to say. I interpreted what they told me to the best of my ability.

I am not an employee of the company nor do I sell their products; I only buy them for myself and to give to the ones I love. And yes, I certainly **take** Calorad®, Agrisept-L®, and some of their other products, and my dogs are on Golden Treat. I'm proud of this book and I feel good about myself for the health it's bringing others.

ACKNOWLEDGMENTS

I have grown to love Jay Sargeant, not only for his passionate speech that motivated me to the point that I couldn't sleep for days thinking of those I could help—IF "*this stuff*" worked—and it has, but Jay is a good person, warm, caring, and sincere. He is a good father, friend, husband and Christian.

I thank Geraldine Heyman, the Director of International Sales and Marketing for Essentially Yours Industries, who had an idea and a plan and built a wondrous team of talented and caring people. She put EYI together.

And to Michel Grisé, the brilliant formulator who introduced products that have enriched the quality of life for countless people—perhaps as many as a few million people or more across the globe. He, too, is warm, caring and dedicated to helping others®.

And Ruby Miller-Lyman; I heard her speak on Calorad®, too. What I learned from Jay, she seconded in her upbeat, flowing style. She's a great motivator, *par excellence*, and I was amazed at her energy, vitality and her work habits. And Donna Green is "Mama Donna" to many.

Then there's Kristan Sargeant, Jay's daughter; what a lovely human being she is as well as another fantastic motivator. The "apple" fell directly under the tree in this instance. And Ann Rogers, who travels the country helping others understand how to use and market Calorad®.

Jim Darechuk (born in Thunder Bay, Canada, now living in Houston) is successful with his business because money is not his main motivating factor; helping others is. I thank his likable and ever smiling partner, Priest Kemper and his wife, Pat who is always at his side; we've become close friends. These three are very special people.

Of the more than 325,000 Independent Distributors in this company, most became involved because Calorad®

worked on them and, like me, they wanted to share their "discovery" with others. The money they can earn is secondary. I am convinced of that.

Essentially Yours Industries is like a prayer by many—answered. They *are* helping mankind! The entire corporate team has produced a kind of magnetism that has carried over into the hearts and souls of their distributors. These are good people doing good things.

The incredible business success of EYI was built on the discovery of Calorad® but I know, deep in my heart, that it's mostly due to the "team" effort and that includes everyone from the top people of the company to the person that uses Calorad®. A product alone, no matter how miraculous, isn't enough. And, the team is ever expanding.

I've found the distributors in this company to be absolutely marvelous, clean-living, caring, Christian people. I've made more friends in the past year than I have in my lifetime. These type of people don't "just happen" to be in this company, they are *drawn* together by a higher power; I'm convinced of that.

People like Rena Davis, Dr. Mark Evans, Dr. Jack Herd and Barbara, Art and Marlyn Burleigh, Dr. Bob DeMaria and Deb, Michael Whelan, Ron Chandler, Marcie and Norman Jackson, Barry Ross, Dr. Brian Brockman, Dave and Bonnie White, John and Marilee Bielski, Dr. Herb Oliver, Vickie Ridge—where on earth have all of you wonderful people been hiding most of my life?

I could go on and on but it's impossible to mention all the remarkable people and the many equally remarkable testimonies I hear each week during my travels. I've flown to 68 cities around the US and Canada in eight months. My second home, now, seems to be Canada. Never have I met a more delightful, friendly COUNTRY of people.

I went when it was cold and, being from the south, it wasn't easy. But, because of people like Gisele and Martin Croteau of Regina, Lucille and Ron Perry of

Saskatoon, Wayne Graham of Edmonton, Tim Blacklock of Kingston, Shawn and Cathy Wootten of Hamilton, Ione Dombrowsky of Calgary, Carol Nickling-Braund, Ontario, and Eliza Fung in Vancouver. I'm going BACK even when the temperature is *colder.*

After spending time with Frank Shaw, Barb Gluck, Maureen and Bernie Gaidosch, and "exploring" in every city (lost) with Wayne Graham, I feel as if I'm part Canadian. I love curling, I don't mind taking my shoes off when I enter a house (or is it hoose?) and it's even helped my punctuation; I only need to work with a *question mark* since all my sentences end with *ey?* My Canadian audiences have averaged 300 to 500 and I feel like a celebrity. Sure I love Canada.

And NEW friends like Don Hyde of Lethridge, Alberta - what an entrepreneur he is - fun to chat with, also. Keith Mason of Victoria B.C., and Denise Akers and Richard Sale of the UK, just wonderful people.

I'm working hard and almost all the time. I love it so much I can't imagine what my life was like before. I'm on a *mission and I must thank you all* for bringing meaning to my life. I'm always available to you - just call.

Calorad® and Essentially Yours Industries and all the people in the company have changed my spiritual life! I feel good about what I'm doing. I like it. I love it. I embrace it.

Pete Billac

And please, after you read this book, give it to someone you truly care for and ask them to do the same.

LOSE FAT WHILE YOU SLEEP
is available through:

Swan Publishing
126 Live Oak
Alvin, TX 77511

(281) 388-2547
Fax (281) 585-3738

or e-mail: swanbooks@ghg.net

Visit our web site at:
http:\\www.swan-pub.com

☆☆*PLEASE HELP US WITH OUR* RESEARCH☆☆

EYI has a new product called **definition**™ *"food for healthy breasts."* This product was designed to help all women who want a proven, safe and healthy way to enhance, shape, tone, firm, uplift and generally perfect the curves of their female form. It can help women who have breast fed their children and whose tissue has been "compromised" from that experience. This **all natural** herbal formula feeds the mammary glands in such a way as to support the muscle structure around them.

We are currently researching this product for a new book. If you have any direct information, quantitative analyses or testimonials about this product, please send your input to the above listed address for Swan Publishing.

ABOUT THE AUTHOR

PETE BILLAC is one of the most sought-after speakers in the United States. He is billed as an Author/Lecturer/Humorist. Pete is a maverick; he writes only what pleases him. He has written 43 full-length books, hundreds of short stories and conducts fun lectures on cruise ships. His topics range from adventure and war, to famous people, history, self-help, health and romance.

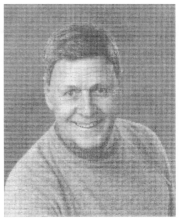

Perhaps you've seen him on Donahue, Sally Jessy Raphael, Good Morning America or any of the other network televison shows. He speaks to Fortune 500 companies on marketing, school kids on reading and writing, and to folks over 60 on keeping physically fit and enjoying life. He makes his audiences laugh . . . hard!

This book, LOSE FAT WHILE YOU SLEEP, is his favorite. His runaway best seller, HOW NOT TO BE LONELY, has sold over 4 million copies. "I feel this will do as well as Lonely," Pete says. "It will absolutely help everyone live a healthier and, hopefully, happier life."

Phil Donahue said, "Pete is an expert at restoring self-confidence and self-esteem in others."

Ken Collins, Syndicated Radio Celebrity Host said, "One of the funniest, most charismatic speakers I have ever heard. He breathes life into every topic. Be sure to attend any function where Pete is featured."